SMOOTHIES FOR ULCERATIVE COLITIS

Nourishing Recipes for Healing and Gut Health

By

Nicole J. Deleon

Copyright

Disclaimer

The information and recipes provided in this Ulcerative Colitis Smoothie Cookbook are intended for informational purposes only. They are not intended as medical advice or as a substitute for professional medical treatment or diagnosis. Always seek the advice of your doctor or other qualified healthcare provider regarding any medical condition or treatment.

The recipes in this cookbook are designed with the dietary considerations of individuals with ulcerative colitis in mind. However, individual needs may vary, and it is important to tailor your diet to your own specific health needs and preferences. It is recommended to consult with a registered dietitian or nutritionist to ensure that the recipes and ingredients are appropriate for your individual dietary requirements and health goals.

The author and publisher of this cookbook make no representations or warranties of any kind, express or implied, about the completeness, accuracy, reliability, suitability, or availability of the information and recipes contained herein. Any reliance you place on such information and recipes is therefore strictly at your own risk.

In no event will the author or publisher be liable for any loss, damage, or injury arising from the use of the information or recipes in this cookbook.

About the author

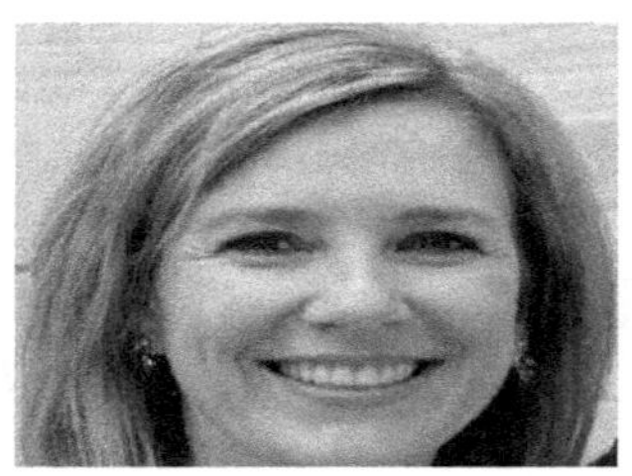

Hello there! I'm Nicole J. Deleon, a passionate health advocate, culinary enthusiast, and wellness coach who is dedicated to helping others attain optimal health through delicious and nutritious meals. My journey with ulcerative colitis has been challenging, but it has also been a source of discovery and empowerment. Through my own experiences, I have learned the amazing healing power of food, and I'm dedicated to helping others find the same relief and joy through nutrition.

Living with ulcerative colitis has given me a first-hand understanding of the daily struggles and triumphs that come with managing a chronic condition. This personal journey encouraged me to dive deeply into the realm of nutrition and culinary arts, seeking natural solutions to control and even reverse symptoms. The result is this collection of smoothie recipes that are easy on the digestive system yet still filled with flavour and vitality.

With a background in nutrition and culinary arts, I bring a unique set of skills to every recipe. My goal is to make smoothies that nourish your body while also bringing joy and fulfilment to your soul. I believe that eating well shouldn't feel like a chore—it should be a delightful and rewarding experience.

In addition to creating this cookbook, I've shared my knowledge through workshops, blogs, and individual coaching session. I appreciate interacting with others and assisting them in gaining control of their digestive health in an enjoyable and fun way. There's nothing more fulfilling than witnessing someone realize that with the correct tools and knowledge, that managing their condition can be both manageable and enjoyable

So, join me on this journey to better health, one delicious smoothie at a time. I'm here to guide you, share tips, and celebrate your successes along the way. Here's to your health, happiness, and many delicious smoothies! Cheers!

Table of contents

INTRODUCTION

Introducing the Ulcerative Smoothie Cookbook, your passport to a journey of delicious relief and digestive wellness! In this vibrant collection, you'll uncover a treasure trove of recipes designed to soothe and nourish, crafted specifically for those managing ulcerative colitis.

Imagine starting your day with a refreshing sunrise smoothie, packed with anti-inflammatory ingredients to gently kick start your morning. Or perhaps you crave a midday pick-me-up that not only satisfies your taste buds but also supports your digestive health with fiber-rich fruits and gut-friendly probiotics.

Each recipe in this cookbook is more than just a blend of ingredients; it's a carefully curated potion of wellness. These smoothies are your go-to choice whether you're looking for a satisfying treat, a quick snack, or a meal replacement. In addition to relieving symptoms, they are made to provide your body with vital nutrients, which will make managing your condition easier and more pleasurable.

With practicable and useful tips on choosing ingredients, blending methods, and nutritional benefits, the Ulcerative Smoothie Cookbook gives you the tools you need to take charge of your health in a deliciously accessible way. Get ready to sip your way to a happier gut and embrace a new chapter of well-being with every sip!

Understanding Ulcerative Colitis

Ulcerative colitis (UC) is a chronic inflammatory bowel disease (IBD) that affects primarily the colon and rectum. It causes inflammation and ulcers in the lining of your large intestine, resulting in symptoms like abdominal pain, diarrhoea, and rectal bleeding. The exact cause of UC is unknown, however it is thought to be the outcome of an abnormal immune reaction that targets the digestive tract. Genetics, environmental factors, and an imbalance in gut bacteria all play a part in its development. Living with UC can be both physically and emotionally challenging. Flare-ups can disrupt your daily routine, and managing the condition often involves significant changes in lifestyle. Diet is an essential part of managing UC since certain foods can cause symptoms while others can help reduce inflammation and promote healing.

The Benefits of Smoothies for Ulcerative Colitis

One of the main challenges in managing UC is ensuring you get the necessary nutrients without aggravating your symptoms. This is where smoothies come in. Smoothies offer a convenient and delicious way to consume a variety of essential nutrients without putting too much strain on your digestive system. Here are some key benefits:

1. **Ease of Digestion:** Smoothies are easy to digest because the blending process breaks down the food into a more easily absorbed form. This is especially beneficial during flare-ups when your digestive system is more sensitive.

2. **Nutrient Density:** Smoothies can be packed with vitamins, minerals, and antioxidants from fruits, vegetables, and other healthy ingredients. This helps ensure you're getting the nutrients your body needs to function properly and support immune health.

3. Hydration: Staying hydrated is crucial for managing UC. Many smoothie recipes include water-rich ingredients like cucumbers, watermelon, and coconut water, which can help you maintain adequate hydration levels.

4. Anti-Inflammatory Properties: Many ingredients commonly used in smoothies, such as berries, leafy greens, ginger, and turmeric, have natural anti-inflammatory properties. Incorporating these into your diet can help reduce inflammation and soothe your digestive tract.

5. Customization: Smoothies are incredibly versatile: You can tailor each recipe to your specific dietary needs, preferences, and the current state of your symptoms. Whether you need a low-fiber option during a flare-up or a high-protein blend for energy, there's a smoothie recipe to suit your needs.

How to Use This Cookbook

This cookbook is organized to make it easy for you to find the perfect smoothie for any occasion. We've divided the recipes into several categories, each designed to address different aspects of managing ulcerative colitis:

1. Breakfast Smoothies: Start your day with energy-boosting blends that are gentle on your digestive system.

2. Anti-Inflammatory Smoothies: Incorporate ingredients that help reduce inflammation and promote gut health.

3. Gut-Healing Smoothies: Focus on ingredients known for their healing properties, such as aloe vera and papaya.

4. High-Protein Smoothies: Ensure you're getting enough protein to maintain muscle mass and support overall health.

5. Calming and Soothing Smoothies: Find blends that can help soothe your digestive system and calm your mind.

6. Immune-Boosting Smoothies: Strengthen your immune system with nutrient-rich ingredients.

7. Low-Fiber Smoothies: Perfect for when you need to reduce fiber intake to prevent irritation.

8. Hydrating Smoothies: Keep your body well-hydrated with water-rich ingredients.

9. Dessert Smoothies: Satisfy your sweet tooth with healthy, gut-friendly options.

Each section includes a variety of recipes, complete with ingredient lists, step-by-step instructions, and tips for customization. We've also included information on the benefits of key ingredients and how they can help manage UC symptoms.

We hope this cookbook inspires you to embrace the power of smoothies in managing your ulcerative colitis. By incorporating these nutrient-packed blends into your daily routine, you can support your digestive health, reduce symptoms, and enjoy delicious, satisfying meals. Here's to better health and happier tummies!

CHAPTER 1: GETTING STARTED

Welcome to the "Getting Started" section of the Ulcerative Colitis Smoothie Cookbook! This section will set you up for success by introducing you to the essential ingredients, equipment, and tips needed to make the most of your smoothie-making experience. Whether you're a smoothie novice or a seasoned pro, these insights will help you create delicious and nutritious blends tailored to your specific needs.

Essential Ingredients and Their Benefits

1. Fruits and Vegetables: Fruits and vegetables are the cornerstone of any great smoothie. They provide a wealth of vitamins, minerals, and antioxidants that support overall health and help reduce inflammation. Berries (like blueberries, strawberries, and raspberries) are packed with antioxidants and anti-inflammatory compounds. Leafy greens (such as spinach and kale) are nutrient-dense and blend well with fruits to create a smooth texture. Bananas and avocados add creaminess and are gentle on the digestive system.

2. Protein Sources: Ensuring adequate protein intake is essential, especially if you are experiencing weight loss or muscle wasting due to UC. Greek yogurt, cottage cheese, and plant-based protein powders (like pea or hemp protein) are excellent additions to your smoothies. They help keep you full and provide the necessary building blocks for tissue repair and immune function.

3. Healthy Fats: Healthy fats are crucial for nutrient absorption and overall health. Adding a tablespoon of nut butter (such as almond or peanut butter), chia seeds, flaxseeds, or avocado can enhance the nutritional profile of your smoothies. These ingredients also add a satisfying texture and flavour.

4. Hydrating Liquids: The liquid base of your smoothie is important for blending and hydration. Coconut water, almond milk, and water are great choices. Coconut water is especially hydrating and rich in electrolytes, while almond milk adds a creamy texture without the lactose that can sometimes aggravate UC symptoms.

5. Anti-Inflammatory Boosters: Certain ingredients have powerful anti-inflammatory properties that can help manage UC symptoms. Ginger and turmeric are two such ingredients. Adding a small piece of fresh ginger or a pinch of turmeric powder to your smoothies can provide significant benefits. Just be mindful of their strong flavours and start with small amounts.

6. Fiber Considerations: While fiber is an essential part of a healthy diet, those with UC need to be cautious. During flare-ups, it may be necessary to reduce fiber intake to avoid irritation. Opt for low-fiber fruits and vegetables like bananas, avocados, and cooked carrots. When you're not experiencing a flare-up, you can gradually incorporate more fiber-rich ingredients like berries, leafy greens, and oats.

Equipment and Tools You Will Need

1. Blender: A high-quality blender is the most important tool for making smoothies. It ensures that all ingredients are well-blended, resulting in a smooth and creamy texture. If you can, invest in a blender with a powerful motor and multiple speed settings. This will help you handle tougher ingredients like frozen fruits and leafy greens with ease.

2. Measuring Cups and Spoons: Accurate measurements help ensure consistency in your recipes. Measuring cups and spoons are essential for portion control, especially when adding potent ingredients like protein powders and spices.

3. Storage Containers: Airtight containers are great for storing pre-made smoothies or leftover ingredients. Mason jars, reusable silicone bags, and glass containers are excellent options. They keep your smoothies fresh and make them easy to grab on the go.

4. Cutting Board and Knife: Preparing your ingredients properly is key to a smooth blending process. A good cutting board and sharp knife will make chopping fruits and vegetables quicker and safer.

Tips for Making the Perfect Smoothie

1. Balance Your Ingredients: A good smoothie has a balance of fruits, vegetables, protein, and healthy fats. This ensures you're getting a well-rounded blend of nutrients. Aim for a mix of sweet and savoury ingredients to create a balanced flavour profile.

2. Start with Liquids: Begin by adding your liquid base to the blender first. This helps the blades move freely and blend the other ingredients more effectively.

3. Layer Your Ingredients: For the best blending results, layer your ingredients starting with the liquids, followed by softer ingredients (like yogurt or nut butter), then fruits and vegetables, and finally ice or frozen items. This order helps prevent clogging and ensures a smooth blend.

4. Blend in Stages: If you're using tough ingredients like kale or frozen fruit, blend in stages. Start at a lower speed to break down the larger pieces, then gradually increase the speed to fully incorporate all ingredients.

5. Taste and Adjust: Don't be afraid to taste your smoothie before pouring it into a glass. If it needs more sweetness, add a bit of honey or a few more pieces of fruit. Add a little more liquid, if it's too thick. Customizing your smoothie to your taste ensures you'll enjoy every sip.

6. Experiment and Have Fun: Smoothie-making is an art and a science. Do not be afraid to experiment with different types of ingredients. You might discover a new favourite blend that perfectly suits your palate and nutritional needs.

By getting started with these foundational tips and tools, you're well on your way to creating delicious, nutritious smoothies that will help you manage your ulcerative colitis effectively. Enjoy the process, and here is to your health and happiness!

CHAPTER 2: BREAKFAST SMOOTHIES

1) Energizing Green Smoothie:

- Prep Time: 5 minutes
- Total Time: 5 minutes
- Servings: 2

INGREDIENTS

- 1 cup spinach
- 1/2 cup kale
- 1 banana
- 1/2 avocado
- 1 cup almond milk
- 1 tablespoon chia seeds
- 1 teaspoon honey (optional)

INSTRUCTIONS

1. Place the almond milk in the blender first.
2. Add the spinach and kale.
3. Peel and add the banana and avocado.
4. Sprinkle in the chia seeds.

5. Add honey for a sweeter taste if desired.

6. Blend on high speed until it's smooth and creamy.

7. Pour into a glass and enjoy immediately.

NUTRITIONAL FACTS

- Calories: 250

- Protein: 5g

- Carbohydrates: 35g

- Fat: 12g

- Fiber: 10g

2) Berry Blast Breakfast Smoothie:

- Prep Time: 5 minutes

- Total time: 5 minutes

- Serving: 2

INGREDIENTS

- 1/2 cup blueberries

- 1/2 cup strawberries, hulled

- 1/2 cup raspberries

- 1/2 cup Greek yogurt

- 1 tablespoon flaxseeds

- 1 cup unsweetened almond milk

- 1/2 cup ice cubes

INSTRUCTIONS

1. Place the almond milk into the blender first.

2. Add the blueberries, strawberries, and raspberries.

3. Add the Greek yogurt and flaxseeds.

4. Add the ice cubes.

5. Blend until it's smooth and creamy on high speed.

6. Serve immediately for a high-fiber, antioxidant-rich treat.

NUTRITIONAL FACTS

- Calories: 190
- Protein: 8g
- Carbohydrates: 30g
- Fat: 5g
- Fiber: 8g

3) Tropical Sunrise Smoothie:

- Prep Time: 5 minutes
- Total time: 5 minutes
- Servings: 2

INGREDIENTS

- 1/2 cup frozen pineapple chunks
- 1/2 cup frozen mango chunks
- 1/2 banana
- 1/2 cup coconut water
- 1/2 cup Greek yogurt
- 1 tablespoon chia seeds
- 1/2 cup ice cubes

INSTRUCTIONS

1. Pour into the blender the coconut water.
2. Add the frozen pineapple chunks, mango chunks, and banana.
3. Add the Greek yogurt and chia seeds.
4. Add the ice cubes.
5. Blend on high speed until it's smooth and creamy.

6. Serve immediately for a refreshing and nutritious start to your day.

NUTRITIONAL FACTS

- Calories: 220
- Protein: 8g
- Carbohydrates: 40g
- Fat: 5g
- Fiber: 6g

4) Oatmeal Cookie Smoothie:

- Prep Time: 5 minutes
- Total time: 5 minutes
- Servings: 2

INGREDIENTS

1. 1 banana
2. 1/4 cup rolled oats
3. 1/2 cup Greek yogurt
4. 1 cup unsweetened almond milk
5. 1 tablespoon almond butter
6. 1 teaspoon honey (optional)
7. 1/2 teaspoon cinnamon
8. 1/2 teaspoon vanilla extract
9. 1/2 cup ice cubes

INSTRUCTIONS

1. Pour into the blender the almond milk.
2. Add the banana, rolled oats, and Greek yogurt.
3. Add the almond butter, honey (if using), cinnamon, and vanilla extract.
4. Add the ice cubes.
5. Blend on high until it is smooth and creamy.

6. Serve immediately for a delicious, dessert-like breakfast smoothie.

NUTRITIONAL FACTS

- Calories: 300
- Protein: 12g
- Carbohydrates: 45g
- Fat: 10g
- Fiber: 6g

CHAPTER 3: ANTI-INFLAMMATORY SMOOTHIES

1) Turmeric and Ginger Smoothie:

- Prep Time: 5 minutes
- Total Time: 5 minutes
- Servings: 2

INGREDIENTS

- 1 cup coconut milk
- 1/2 banana
- 1 teaspoon turmeric powder
- 1/2 teaspoon fresh ginger, grated
- 1/2 teaspoon cinnamon
- 1 tablespoon honey (optional)
- 1/2 cup ice cubes

INSTRUCTION

1. Pour into the blender the coconut milk.

2. Add the banana, turmeric powder, grated ginger, and cinnamon.

3. Add honey for a sweeter taste if desired.

4. Add the ice cubes.

5. Blend on high speed until it is smooth and well-combined.

6. Serve immediately for a refreshing, anti-inflammatory drink.

NUTRITIONAL FACTS

- Calories: 180
- Protein: 2g
- Carbohydrates: 35g
- Fat: 6g
- Fiber: 4g

2) Blueberry Antioxidant Smoothie:

- Prep Time: 5 minutes
- Total Time: 5 minutes
- Servings: 2

INGREDIENTS

- 1 cup blueberries (fresh or frozen)
- 1/2 cup Greek yogurt
- 1/2 banana
- 1 tablespoon flaxseeds
- 1 cup unsweetened almond milk
- 1/2 cup ice cubes

INSTRUCTIONS

1. Pour into the blender the almond milk.
2. Add the blueberries, Greek yogurt, and banana.
3. Add the flaxseeds.
4. Add the ice cubes.
5. Blend on high speed until it is smooth and creamy.
6. Serve immediately for a powerful antioxidant boost.

NUTRITIONAL FACTS

- Calories: 200

- Protein: 8g

- Carbohydrates: 30g

- Fat: 6g

- Fiber: 6g

3) Pineapple and Spinach Smoothie:

- Prep Time: 5 minutes
- Total Time: 5 minutes
- Servings: 2

INGREDIENTS

- 1 cup fresh pineapple chunks
- 1 cup spinach
- 1/2 banana
- 1/2 cup Greek yogurt
- 1 cup coconut water
- 1 tablespoon chia seeds
- 1/2 cup ice cubes

INSTRUCTIONS

1. Pour into the blender the coconut water.
2. Add the pineapple chunks, spinach, and banana.
3. Add the Greek yogurt and chia seeds.
4. Add the ice cubes.
5. Blend on high speed until it is smooth and well-combined.

6. Serve immediately for a nutrient-rich green smoothie.

NUTRITIONAL FACTS

- Calories: 210
- Protein: 9g
- Carbohydrates: 35g
- Fat: 4g
- Fiber: 5g

4) Cherry Almond Smoothie:

- Prep Time: 5 minutes
- Total Time: 5 minutes
- Servings: 2

INGREDIENTS

- 1 cup frozen cherries
- 1/2 cup unsweetened almond milk
- 1/2 cup Greek yogurt
- 1 tablespoon almond butter
- 1 teaspoon honey (optional)
- 1/2 cup ice cubes

INSTRUCTIONS

1. Pour into the blender the almond milk.
2. Add the frozen cherries, Greek yogurt, and almond butter.
3. Add honey for a sweeter taste if desired.
4. Add the ice cubes.
5. Blend on high speed until it is smooth and creamy.
6. Serve immediately.

NUTRITIONAL FACTS

- Calories: 220
- Protein: 10g
- Carbohydrates: 25g
- Fat: 10g
- Fiber: 4g

CHAPTER 4: GUT-HEALING SMOOTHIES

1) Carrot and Ginger Smoothie:

- Prep Time: 10 minutes
- Total Time: 10 minutes
- Servings: 2

INGREDIENTS

- 1 cup carrots, peeled and chopped
- 1/2 banana
- 1/2 teaspoon fresh ginger, grated
- 1/2 cup orange juice
- 1/2 cup Greek yogurt
- 1 tablespoon honey (optional)
- 1/2 cup ice cubes

INSTRUCTIONS

1. Pour into the blender the orange juice.
2. Add the chopped carrots, banana, and grated ginger.
3. Add the Greek yogurt.
4. Add honey if you prefer a sweeter taste.

5. Add the ice cubes.

6. Blend on high speed until it is smooth and creamy.

7. Serve immediately for a refreshing and energizing smoothie.

NUTRITIONAL FACTS

- Calories: 190
- Protein: 6g
- Carbohydrates: 35g
- Fat: 3g
- Fiber: 4g

2) Aloe Vera and Cucumber Smoothie:

- Prep Time: 10 minutes
- Total Time: 10 minutes
- Servings: 2

INGREDIENTS

- 1/2 cup fresh aloe vera gel
- 1 cucumber, peeled and chopped
- 1/2 cup coconut water
- 1 tablespoon lemon juice
- 1 teaspoon honey (optional)
- 1/2 cup ice cubes

INSTRUCTIONS

1. . Pour into the blender the coconut water.
2. Add the aloe vera gel, chopped cucumber, and lemon juice.
3. Add honey if desired.
4. Add the ice cubes.
5. Blend on high speed until it is smooth.
6. Serve immediately.

NUTRITIONAL FACTS

- Calories: 70

- Protein: 1g

- Carbohydrates: 15g

- Fat: 0g

- Fiber: 3g

3) Papaya Digestive Smoothie:

- Prep Time: 5 minutes
- Total Time: 5 minutes
- Servings: 2

INGREDIENTS

- 1 cup of ripe peeled and cubed papaya
- 1/2 banana
- 1/2 cup Greek yogurt
- 1/2 cup coconut water
- 1 teaspoon fresh ginger, grated
- 1/2 cup ice cubes

INSTRUCTIONS

1. Pour into the blender the coconut water.
2. Add the papaya, banana, Greek yogurt, and grated ginger.
3. Add the ice cubes.
4. Blend on high speed until it is smooth and creamy.
5. Serve immediately.

NUTRITIONAL FACTS

- Calories: 160
- Protein: 6g
- Carbohydrates: 30g
- Fat: 2g
- Fiber: 4g

4) Banana and Yogurt Smoothie:

- Prep Time: 5 minutes
- Cook Time: 5 minutes
- Servings: 2

INGREDIENTS

- 1 banana
- 1/2 cup Greek yogurt
- 1 cup unsweetened almond milk
- 1 tablespoon honey
- 1/2 teaspoon vanilla extract
- 1/2 cup ice cubes

INSTRUCTIONS

1. Pour into the blender the almond milk.
2. Add the banana, Greek yogurt, honey, and vanilla extract.
3. Add the ice cubes.
4. Blend on high speed until it is smooth and creamy.
5. Serve immediately.

NUTRITIONAL FACTS

- Calories: 200

- Protein: 8g

- Carbohydrates: 35g

- Fat: 4g

- Fiber: 3g

CHAPTER 5:

HIGH-PROTEIN SMOOTHIES

1) Peanut Butter Banana Smoothie:

- Prep Time: 5 minutes
- Total Time: 5 minutes
- Servings: 2

INGREDIENTS

- 1 banana
- 2 tablespoons peanut butter
- 1 cup unsweetened almond milk
- 1/2 teaspoon cinnamon
- 1/2 teaspoon vanilla extract
- 1/2 cup ice cubes

INSTRUCTIONS

1. Pour into the blender the almond milk.
2. Add the banana and peanut butter.
3. Add the cinnamon and vanilla extract.

4. Add the ice cubes.

5. Blend on high speed until it is smooth and creamy.

6. Serve immediately.

NUTRITIONAL FACTS

- Calories: 300

- Protein: 8g

- Carbohydrates: 35g

- Fat: 14g

- Fiber: 5g

2) Chocolate Avocado Smoothie:

- Prep Time: 5 minutes
- Total Time: 5 minutes
- Servings: 2

INGREDIENTS

- 1/2 avocado
- 1 banana
- 1 cup unsweetened almond milk
- 1 tablespoon cocoa powder
- 1 tablespoon honey
- 1/2 cup ice cubes

INSTRUCTIONS

1. Pour into the blender the almond milk.
2. Add the avocado, banana, cocoa powder, and honey.
3. Add the ice cubes.
4. Blend on high speed until it is smooth and creamy.
5. Serve immediately.

NUTRITIONAL FACTS

- Calories: 260

- Protein: 4g

- Carbohydrates: 40g

- Fat: 10g

- Fiber: 8g

3) Almond Butter and Berry Smoothie:

- Prep Time: 5 minutes
- Total Time: 5 minutes
- Servings: 2

INGREDIENTS

- 1/2 cup blueberries
- 1/2 cup strawberries, hulled
- 1 tablespoon almond butter
- 1 cup unsweetened almond milk
- 1/2 cup Greek yogurt
- 1/2 cup ice cubes

INSTRUCTIONS

1. Pour into the blender the almond milk.
2. Add the blueberries, strawberries, almond butter, and Greek yogurt.
3. Add the ice cubes.
4. Blend on high speed until it's smooth and creamy.
5. Serve immediately.

NUTRITIONAL FACTS

- Calories: 230
- Protein: 10g
- Carbohydrates: 30g
- Fat: 8g
- Fiber: 5g

4) Hemp Protein Smoothie:

- Prep Time: 5 minutes
- Total Time: 5 minutes
- Servings: 2

INGREDIENTS

- 1 scoop hemp protein powder
- 1 banana
- 1 cup unsweetened almond milk
- 1 tablespoon honey
- 1/2 teaspoon vanilla extract
- 1/2 cup ice cubes

INSTRUCTIONS

1. Fill the blender with the almond milk.
2. Add the hemp protein powder, banana, honey, and vanilla extract.
3. Add the ice cubes.
4. Blend on high speed until it is smooth and creamy.
5. Serve immediately.

NUTRITIONAL FACTS

- Calories: 200
- Protein: 15g
- Carbohydrates: 25g
- Fat: 6g
- Fber: 5g

CHAPTER 6: CALMING AND SOOTHING SMOOTHIES

1) Chamomile and Honey Smoothie:

- Prep Time: 10 minutes
- Total Time: 10 minutes
- Servings: 2

INGREDIENTS

- 1 cup brewed chamomile tea, cooled
- 1 banana
- 1/2 cup Greek yogurt
- 1 tablespoon honey
- 1/2 teaspoon vanilla extract
- 1/2 cup ice cubes

INSTRUCTIONS

1. Pour into the blender the cooled chamomile tea.
2. Add the banana, Greek yogurt, honey, and vanilla extract.
3. Add the ice cubes.

4. Blend at a high speed until the mixture is smooth and creamy.

5. Serve immediately.

NUTRITIONAL FACTS

- Calories: 160
- Protein: 6g
- Carbohydrates: 30g
- Fat: 2g
- Fiber: 3g

2) Lavender Blueberry Smoothie:

- Prep Time: 10 minutes
- Total Time: 10 minutes
- Servings: 2

INGREDIENTS

- 1/2 cup blueberries
- 1 cup unsweetened almond milk
- 1/2 cup Greek yogurt
- 1 teaspoon dried lavender buds
- 1 tablespoon honey
- 1/2 cup ice cubes

INSTRUCTIONS

1. Pour into the blender the almond milk.
2. Add the blueberries, Greek yogurt, dried lavender buds, and honey.
3. Add the ice cubes.
4. Blend on high speed until it is smooth and creamy.
5. Serve immediately.

NUTRITIONAL FACTS

- Calories: 170
- Protein: 8g
- Carbohydrates: 28g
- Fat: 4g
- Fiber: 4g

3) Melon Mint Smoothie:

- Prep Time: 5 minutes
- Total Time: 5 minutes
- Servings: 2

INGREDIENTS

- 1 cup cantaloupe, cubed
- 1/2 cup honeydew melon, cubed
- 1/2 cup Greek yogurt
- 1/2 cup coconut water
- 1 tablespoon fresh mint leaves
- 1/2 cup ice cubes

INSTRUCTIONS

1. Pour into the blender the coconut water.
2. Add the cantaloupe, honeydew melon, Greek yogurt, and mint leaves.
3. Add the ice cubes.
4. Blend at a high speed until the mixture is smooth and creamy.
5. Serve immediately.

NUTRITIONAL FACTS

- Calories: 150
- Protein: 6g
- Carbohydrates: 28g
- Fat: 3g
- Fiber: 3g

4) Coconut Water and Mango Smoothie:

- Prep Time: 5 minutes
- Total Time: 5 minutes
- Servings: 2

INGREDIENTS

- 1 cup frozen mango chunks
- 1 cup coconut water
- 1/2 banana
- 1/2 cup Greek yogurt
- 1 tablespoon chia seeds
- 1/2 cup ice cubes

INSTRUCTIONS

1. Pour into the blender the coconut water.
2. Add the mango chunks, banana, Greek yogurt, and chia seeds.
3. Add the ice cubes.
4. Blend at a high speed until the mixture is smooth and creamy.
5. Serve immediately.

NUTRITIONAL FACTS

- Calories: 210
- Protein: 8g
- Carbohydrates: 40g
- Fat: 3g
- Fiber: 5g

CHAPTER 7:
IMMUNE-BOOSTING SMOOTHIES

1) Citrus Immunity Smoothie:

- Prep Time: 5 minutes
- Total Time: 5minutes
- Servings: 2

INGREDIENTS

- 1 orange, peeled and segmented
- 1/2 grapefruit, peeled and segmented
- 1/2 lemon, juiced
- 1/2 cup Greek yogurt
- 1 tablespoon honey
- 1/2 cup ice cubes

INSTRUCTIONS

1. Add the orange, grapefruit, and lemon juice to the blender.
2. Add the Greek yogurt and honey.
3. Add the ice cubes.

4. Blend on high speed it is smooth and creamy.

5. Serve immediately.

NUTRITIONAL FACTS

- Calories: 180

- Protein: 6g

- Carbohydrates: 38g

- Fat: 2g

- Fiber: 4g

2) Kiwi and Strawberry Smoothie:

- Prep Time: 5 minutes
- Total Time: 5 minutes
- Servings: 2

INGREDIENTS

- 1 kiwi, peeled and sliced
- 1/2 cup strawberries, hulled
- 1/2 banana
- 1/2 cup Greek yogurt
- 1 cup unsweetened almond milk
- 1 tablespoon honey (optional)
- 1/2 cup ice cubes

INSTRUCTIONS

- Pour into the blender the almond milk.
- Add the kiwi, strawberries, banana, and Greek yogurt.
- Add honey for a sweeter taste if desired.
- Add the ice cubes.
- Blend on high speed it is smooth and creamy.
- Serve immediately.

NUTRITIONAL FACTS

- Calories: 190
- Protein: 8g
- Carbohydrates: 34g
- Fat: 4g
- Fiber: 5g

3) Recipe: Beetroot and Apple Smoothie:

- Prep Time: 10 minutes
- Total Time: 10 minutes
- Servings: 2

INGREDIENTS

- 1 small beetroot, peeled and chopped
- 1 apple, cored and chopped
- 1/2 banana
- 1/2 cup Greek yogurt
- 1 cup unsweetened almond milk
- 1 tablespoon honey (optional)
- 1/2 cup ice cubes

INSTRUCTIONS

1. Pour into the blender the almond milk.
2. Add the beetroot, apple, banana, and Greek yogurt.
3. Add honey if desired.
4. Add the ice cubes.
5. Blend on high speed it is smooth and creamy.
6. Serve immediately.

NUTRITIONAL FACTS

- Calories: 200

- Protein: 8g

- Carbohydrates: 40g

- Fat: 3g

- Fiber: 6g

4) Green Apple and Kale Smoothie:

- Prep Time: 5 minutes
- Total Time: 5 minutes
- Servings: 2

INGREDIENTS

- 1 green apple, cored and chopped
- 1 cup kale, stems removed
- 1/2 banana
- 1/2 cup Greek yogurt
- 1 cup unsweetened almond milk
- 1 tablespoon honey (optional)
- 1/2 cup ice cubes

INSTRUCTIONS

- Pour into the blender the almond milk.
- Add the green apple, kale, banana, and Greek yogurt.
- Add honey if desired.
- Add the ice cubes.
- Blend on high speed until it is smooth and creamy.
- Serve immediately.

NUTRITIONAL FACTS

- Calories: 210

- Protein: 9g

- Carbohydrates: 38g

- Fat: 4g

- Fiber: 7g

CHAPTER 8: LOW-FIBER SMOOTHIES

1) Smooth Banana Smoothie:

- Prep Time: 5 minutes
- Total Time: 5 minutes
- Servings: 2

INGREDIENTS

- 1 banana
- 1/2 cup Greek yogurt
- 1 cup unsweetened almond milk
- 1 tablespoon honey
- 1/2 teaspoon vanilla extract
- 1/2 cup ice cubes

INSTRUCTIONS

1. Pour into the blender the almond milk.
2. Add the banana, Greek yogurt, honey, and vanilla extract.
3. Add the ice cubes.
4. Blend on high speed until it is smooth and creamy.

5. Serve immediately.

NUTRITIONAL FACTS

- Calories: 200
- Protein: 8g
- Carbohydrates: 35g
- Fat: 4g
- Fiber: 3g

2) Cucumber Melon Smoothie:

- Prep Time: 5 minutes

- Total Time: 5 minutes

- Servings: 2

INGREDIENTS

- 1 cucumber, peeled and chopped

- 1 cup honeydew melon, cubed

- 1/2 cup Greek yogurt

- 1 cup coconut water

- 1 tablespoon fresh mint leaves

- 1/2 cup ice cubes

INSTRUCTIONS

1. Pour into the blender the coconut water.

2. Add the cucumber, honeydew melon, Greek yogurt, and mint leaves.

3. Add the ice cubes.

4. Blend on high speed until it is smooth and creamy.

5. Serve immediately.

NUTRITIONAL FACTS

- Calories: 140
- Protein: 6g
- Carbohydrates: 26g
- Fat: 3g
- Fiber: 3g

3) Simple Pear Smoothie:

- Prep Time: 5 minutes

- Total Time: 5 minutes

- Servings: 2

INGREDIENTS

- 1 pear, cored and chopped

- 1/2 banana

- 1/2 cup Greek yogurt

- 1 cup unsweetened almond milk

- 1 tablespoon honey (optional)

- 1/2 teaspoon cinnamon

- 1/2 cup ice cubes

INSTRUCTIONS

1. Pour into the blender the almond milk.

2. Add the pear, banana, Greek yogurt, honey, and cinnamon.

3. Add the ice cubes.

4. Blend on high speed until it is smooth and creamy.

5. Serve immediately.

NUTRITIONAL FACTS

- Calories: 190
- Protein: 8g
- Carbohydrates: 35g
- Fat: 3g
- Fiber: 5g

4) Creamy Pumpkin Smoothie:

- Prep Time: 5 minutes
- Total Time: 5 minutes
- Servings: 2

INGREDIENTS

- 1/2 cup pumpkin puree
- 1/2 banana
- 1/2 cup Greek yogurt
- 1 cup unsweetened almond milk
- 1 tablespoon maple syrup
- 1/2 teaspoon pumpkin pie spice
- 1/2 cup ice cubes

INSTRUCTIONS

- Pour into the blender the almond milk.
- Add the pumpkin puree, banana, Greek yogurt, maple syrup, and pumpkin pie spice.
- Add the ice cubes.
- Blend on high speed until it is smooth and creamy.
- Serve immediately.

NUTRITIONAL FACTS

- Calories: 180
- Protein: 8g
- Carbohydrates: 30g
- Fat: 3g
- Fiber: 4g

CHAPTER 9: HYDRATING SMOOTHIES

1) Watermelon Cooler Smoothie:

- Prep Time: 5 minutes
- Total Time: 5minutes
- Servings: 2

INGREDIENTS

- 1 cup watermelon, cubed and seeds removed
- 1/2 cup cucumber, peeled and chopped
- 1/2 cup Greek yogurt
- 1 cup coconut water
- 1 tablespoon lime juice
- 1/2 cup ice cubes

INSTRUCTIONS

1. Pour into the blender the coconut water.
2. Add the watermelon, cucumber, Greek yogurt, and lime juice.
3. Add the ice cubes.
4. Blend on high speed until it is smooth and creamy.

5. Serve immediately.

NUTRITIONAL FACTS

- Calories: 120
- Protein: 6g
- Carbohydrates: 20g
- Fat: 2g
- Fiber: 2g

2) Cucumber and Lime Smoothie:

- Prep Time: 5 minutes

- Total Time: 5 minutes

- Servings: 2

INGREDIENTS

- 1 cucumber, peeled and chopped

- 1/2 lime, juiced

- 1/2 cup Greek yogurt

- 1 cup coconut water

- 1 tablespoon honey

- 1/2 cup ice cubes

INSTRUCTIONS

1. Pour into the blender the coconut water.

2. Add the cucumber, lime juice, Greek yogurt, and honey.

3. Add the ice cubes.

4. Blend on high speed until it is smooth and creamy.

5. Serve immediately.

NUTRITIONAL FACTS

- Calories: 110
- Protein: 6g
- Carbohydrates: 20g
- Fat: 2g
- Fiber: 2g

3) Aloe Coconut Water Smoothie:

- Prep Time: 10 minutes
- Total Time: 10 minutes
- Servings: 2

INGREDIENTS

- 1/2 cup fresh aloe vera gel
- 1 cup coconut water
- 1/2 cup pineapple, cubed
- 1 tablespoon honey
- 1/2 cup ice cubes

INSTRUCTIONS

1. Pour into the blender the coconut water.
2. Add the aloe vera gel, pineapple, and honey.
3. Add the ice cubes.
4. Blend on high speed until it is smooth and creamy.
5. Serve immediately.

NUTRITIONAL FACTS

- Calories: 90
- Protein: 1g
- Carbohydrates: 22g
- Fat: 0g
- Fiber: 3g

4) Pineapple Coconut Smoothie:

- Prep Time: 5 minutes
- Total Time: 5 minutes
- Servings: 2

INGREDIENTS

- 1 cup pineapple chunks
- 1/2 cup coconut milk
- 1/2 banana
- 1/2 cup Greek yogurt
- 1 tablespoon honey (optional)
- 1/2 cup ice cubes

INSTRUCTIONS

1. Pour into the blender the coconut water.
2. Add the pineapple chunks, banana, Greek yogurt, and honey.
3. Add the ice cubes.
4. Blend on high speed until it is smooth and creamy.
5. Serve immediately.

NUTRITIONAL FACTS

- Calories: 210
- Protein: 6g
- Carbohydrates: 35g
- Fat: 7g
- Fiber: 3g

CHAPTER 10: DESSERT SMOOTHIES

1) Chocolate Banana Smoothie:

- Prep Time: 5 minutes
- Total Time: 5 minutes
- Servings: 2

INGREDIENTS

- 1 banana
- 1 tablespoon cocoa powder
- 1 cup unsweetened almond milk
- 1/2 cup Greek yogurt
- 1 tablespoon honey
- 1/2 teaspoon vanilla extract
- 1/2 cup ice cubes

INSTRUCTIONS

1. Pour the almond milk into the blender.
2. Add the banana, cocoa powder, Greek yogurt, honey, and vanilla extract.

3. Add the ice cubes.

4. Blend on high speed until it is smooth and creamy.

5. Serve immediately.

NUTRITIONAL FACTS

- Calories: 200

- Protein: 8g

- Carbohydrates: 35g

- Fat: 4g

- Fiber: 5g

2) Coconut Cream Pie Smoothie:

- Prep Time: 5 minutes
- Total Time: 5 minutes
- Servings: 2

INGREDIENTS

- 1/2 cup coconut milk
- 1/2 cup Greek yogurt
- 1 banana
- 1 tablespoon shredded coconut
- 1 tablespoon honey
- 1/2 teaspoon vanilla extract
- 1/2 cup ice cubes

INSTRUCTIONS

1. Pour the coconut milk into the blender.
2. Add the Greek yogurt, banana, shredded coconut, honey, and vanilla extract.
3. Add the ice cubes.
4. Blend on high speed until it is smooth and creamy.
5. Serve immediately.

NUTRITIONAL FACTS

- Calories: 230
- Protein: 8g
- Carbohydrates: 32g
- Fat: 9g
- Fiber: 4g

3) Strawberry Shortcake Smoothie:

- Prep Time: 5 minutes
- Total Time: 5 minutes
- Servings: 2

INGREDIENTS

- 1 cup strawberries, hulled
- 1/2 cup Greek yogurt
- 1 cup unsweetened almond milk
- 1 tablespoon honey
- 1/2 teaspoon vanilla extract
- 1/2 cup ice cubes

INSTRUCTIONS

1. Pour the almond milk into the blender.
2. Add the strawberries, Greek yogurt, honey, and vanilla extract.
3. Add the ice cubes.
4. Blend on high speed until it is smooth and creamy.
5. Serve immediately.

NUTRITIONAL FACTS

- Calories: 180
- Protein: 8g
- Carbohydrates: 30g
- Sugars: 22g
- Fat: 4g
- Fiber: 4g

4) Vanilla Peach Smoothie:

- Prep Time: 5 minutes
- Total Time: 5 minutes
- Servings: 2

INGREDIENTS

- 1 peach, pitted and sliced
- 1/2 banana
- 1/2 cup Greek yogurt
- 1 cup unsweetened almond milk
- 1/2 teaspoon vanilla extract
- 1 tablespoon honey (optional)
- 1/2 cup ice cubes

INSTRUCTIONS

1. Pour the almond milk into the blender.
2. Add the peach, banana, Greek yogurt, vanilla extract, and honey.
3. Add the ice cubes.
4. Blend on high speed until it is smooth and creamy.
5. Serve immediately.

NUTRITIONAL FACTS

- Calories: 190
- Protein: 8g
- Carbohydrates: 32g
- Fat: 4g
- Fiber: 3g

CHAPTER 11: TIPS FOR PERSONALIZING YOUR SMOOTHIES

1. Adjusting Sweetness:

Finding the right level of sweetness for your smoothie is crucial for enjoying your drink. Natural sweeteners like honey, maple syrup, agave nectar, or dates can add the perfect touch of sweetness without the need for refined sugars. If you prefer to use fruit as your sweetener, opt for naturally sweet fruits like bananas, mangoes, or pineapples. If you're looking to reduce the sugar content, use low-sugar fruits such as berries, cucumbers, or green apples. Remember, the ripeness of the fruit also affects the sweetness, so adjust accordingly.

2. Enhancing Creaminess:

For a luxuriously creamy smoothie, incorporate ingredients like Greek yogurt, avocado, or silken tofu. These additions not only improve texture but also boost the nutritional content. For those avoiding dairy, alternatives like coconut milk, almond milk, or oat milk provide a creamy base without compromising on taste. Soaked nuts such as cashews or almonds can also be blended to create a smooth, rich texture.

3. Boosting Nutrition:

Make your smoothies more nutrient-dense by adding leafy greens like spinach, kale, or Swiss chard. These greens blend well and are almost tasteless when mixed with fruits. Super foods like chia seeds, flaxseeds, hemp seeds, or spirulina can be sprinkled in for additional vitamins, minerals, and omega-3 fatty acids. If you need more protein, consider adding protein powders such as whey, pea, or soy protein.

4. Experimenting with Flavours:

Don't hesitate to experiment with different flavours. Spices like cinnamon, nutmeg, ginger, or turmeric can provide a warm and exotic twist. Fresh herbs like mint, basil, or cilantro can give your smoothie a refreshing and unique taste. Flavour extracts such as vanilla, almond, or coconut can further enhance your smoothie's flavour profile.

5. Texture Adjustments:

The texture of your smoothie can make a big difference in your enjoyment. For a thicker smoothie, add more frozen fruits, yogurt, or ice cubes. If you find your smoothie too thick, thin it out with water, coconut water, or additional milk. Blending longer will result in a smoother texture, while pulsing the blender can give a chunkier consistency if preferred.

6. Adding Healthy Fats:

Healthy fats are essential for satiety and overall health. Nut butters like peanut, almond, or cashew butter can add richness and flavour to your smoothie. A small amount of coconut oil or flaxseed oil can also boost the nutritional content. Avocado is another great option that adds creaminess without overpowering the taste.

7. Experimenting with Bases:

The liquid base of your smoothie greatly influences its taste and nutritional content. Instead of sticking to just one type of liquid, try different bases like coconut water, green tea, herbal tea, or various fruit juices. Mixing and matching these bases can help you find your preferred flavour and nutritional profile.

8. Including Vegetables:

Vegetables can add a nutritional punch to your smoothies. Carrots, beets, or cucumbers are great options for added vitamins and minerals. For a neutral flavour and creamy texture, try adding steamed and cooled cauliflower or zucchini. These veggies blend well and don't alter the taste significantly.

8) Customizing for Dietary Needs:

Personalize your smoothies to fit your dietary requirements. For vegan smoothies, use plant-based yogurts and milks. For keto or low-carb options, use low-carb fruits like berries, avocados, and unsweetened almond milk. Ensure all added ingredients are certified gluten-free if you have a gluten intolerance.

9. Adding Unique Ingredients:

Take your smoothies to the next level with unique ingredients like matcha powder, acai powder, or maca powder. These super foods not only offer unique flavour but also provide various health benefits. Cooked and cooled grains like quinoa or oats can add fiber and texture. A splash of apple cider vinegar or lemon juice can give a tangy kick and aid digestion.

10. Seasonal and Local Ingredients:

Using seasonal fruits and vegetables ensures you get the freshest and most flavourful ingredients. Supporting local farmers by incorporating locally grown produce not only benefits your health but also the community. Seasonal ingredients can inspire new smoothie combinations and keep your smoothie routine exciting.

11. Balancing Your Smoothie:

Aim for a balanced mix of carbohydrates (fruits), proteins (yogurt, protein powder), and fats (nuts, seeds) to create a complete meal in a glass. This balance ensures you get the necessary nutrients to keep you energized throughout the day. Adjust ingredients based on your nutritional goals and taste preferences to create your perfect smoothie.

By following these tips, you can personalize your smoothies to suit your taste and dietary needs, making each smoothie a delightful and nutritious experience.

CONCLUSION

Congratulations on reaching the end of the Ulcerative Colitis Smoothie Cookbook! This journey through vibrant flavours and nutrient-packed ingredients is intended to not only satisfy your taste buds, but also to benefit your health in significant ways. Each smoothie recipe in this book has been carefully created to help you manage ulcerative colitis while also enjoying tasty, satisfying meals.

Living with ulcerative colitis can present its challenges, but your diet doesn't have to be one of them. By embracing these smoothie recipes, you've taken a huge step toward making your dietary choices a source of pleasure and healing. Each ingredient has been selected for its soothing, anti-inflammatory effects, so that every sip helps to calm your digestive system and promote general well-being.

We hope you've found joy in the simplicity and ease of these recipes. Smoothies are not just a quick fix; they are a versatile tool for integrating more fruits, vegetables, and super foods into your diet. Whether you start your day with a refreshing Tropical Sunrise Smoothie, boost your midday energy with a nutrient-dense Green Apple and Kale Smoothie, or wind down with a calming Chamomile and Honey Smoothie, you're making choices that honour your body's needs.

Remember, the journey to managing ulcerative colitis is unique for everyone. These smoothies offer a foundation, but feel free to personalize them to suit your taste preferences and nutritional goals. Add your favourite fruits, experiment with different greens, or sprinkle in some extra super foods. The flexibility of smoothies means you can continually adapt and enjoy them without getting bored.

As you continue on your health journey, consider the broader implications of your dietary choices. Proper nutrition can dramatically improve your quality of life by increasing your energy, mood, and general sense of well-being. These smoothies are more than simply recipes; they demonstrate the power of food as medicine, providing an enjoyable way to improve your health from the inside out. So here's to you, to your health, and to the many delightful smoothies you'll enjoy from this book. May each blend bring you closer to a happier, healthier you.

Cheers to sipping your way to wellness, one smoothie at a time. Enjoy every delicious moment, and remember that you're not just nourishing your body, but also nurturing your journey towards a more vibrant and balanced life.

REVIEW

Hey there!

I hope this message finds you well. We'd love to hear your thoughts on Smoothies for Ulcerative Colitis.

Your feedback is extremely valuable to us! We want to know about your experience, whether you tried just one recipe or the entire cookbook. Your insights helps us learn what works and where we can improve to better support your health and culinary adventures.

Your feedback is very important to us. Please reach out and share your opinions. Together, we can make healthy and delicious choices a part of our daily lives. Thank you for being a part of our community and choosing to prioritize your health with us. Here's too many more smoothie-filled adventures!

9 7 9 8 3 3 2 8 9 3 5 5 1